THE LITT
GYM
ETIQUETTE

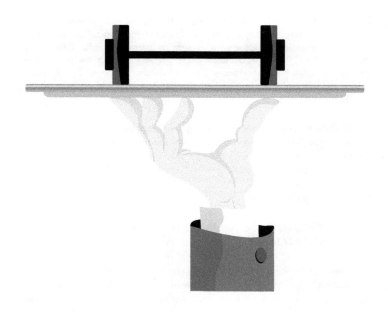

A HANDBOOK FOR DEALING WITH
ANNOYING PEOPLE AT THE GYM

LORI L. PINES

The Little Book of Gym Etiquette

A Handbook for Dealing with Annoying People at the Gym

By Lori L. Pines
Conifer Press

Published by Conifer Press, Austin, TX 78717
Copyright ©2013 Lori L. Pines
All rights reserved.

Cover Design: Bella Guzmán, www.highwirecreative.com
Interior Page Design: Davis Creative, www.daviscreative.com
Illustrations: Jerry McCabe
                Edmond Agalliu
                Lori L. Pines
                Ashley Smith

Library of Congress Control Number: 2011945695
ISBN: 978-0-9847108-0-5

Quantity discounts are available on bulk purchases of this book for educational, gift purposes, or as membership/subscription premiums. Special books or book excerpts can also be created to fit specific needs. For information, please contact Conifer Press, PO Box 170627, Austin, TX 78717 ph: 512-250-8546

The Little Book of Gym Etiquette

A Handbook for Dealing with
Annoying People at the Gym

By Lori L. Pines

To my family for encouraging me to work out, and to Edi, my favorite trainer.

Why
We Need
Gym Etiquette

We are all supposed to get a lot of exercise. For many people, the best place to do that is at a public gym. But, let's face facts—it isn't easy getting to the gym. You have to walk or drive there, change your clothes, psych yourself up for the pain and exertion, and then clean yourself up and change your clothes afterwards. The very last thing we need is a further deterrent to getting to the gym. That is why there is nothing more infuriatingly annoying than having to deal with people who don't know how to behave there. Those are the people who simply have no gym etiquette, and who end up (intentionally or unintentionally) evoking "gym rage" in others, i.e., the strong desire to strangle, push out a window, or otherwise do bodily harm to a person working out nearby.

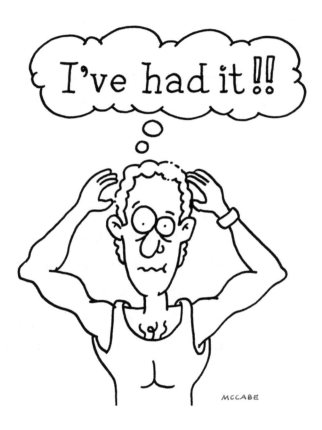

Despite the hassle involved in getting to the gym, working out is supposed to be a stress-relieving, not stress-inducing activity. Therefore, it is of utmost importance that we do everything we possibly can to enable all gym-goers to get the most out of each workout and to minimize those uncomfortable and distracting feelings of gym rage. In this book, I'm going to identify what might be causing your gym rage, help you know what to say to encourage offending gym-goers to change their behavior, and give you some tips for dealing with them if they don't.

To make working out a more pleasurable experience for everyone, all gym-goers should observe some simple rules of gym etiquette. That is what this guide is all about—to set forth, once and for all, the unwritten rules of working out in a public gym. The goal is for all of us to do what so many gym receptionists and cardio machines implore us to do: to "have a good workout."

The six essential rules of gym etiquette (and sub-rules) detailed in this guide remind everyone to avoid being any of the following at the gym:

A slob:
a messy/disgusting gym-goer

A hog:
a selfish gym-goer

A space invader:
a gym-goer who has no respect
for the personal space of others

A super-talker:

an annoying chatterbox of a gym-goer

A grouch:

a miserable, unfriendly,
or impolite gym-goer

An exhibitionist:

a gym-goer who either
intentionally or unintentionally
shows us more of his or her body
than we ever need or care to see

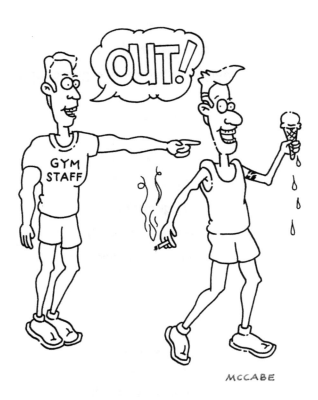

These are the rules of the gym that every single gym-goer should review before ever setting foot in one—and that every gym-goer should be required to follow. (And, if I had my way, gym-goers who refuse to do so would, after proper warning, be banned from working out in the presence of others—and perhaps even evicted by gym bouncers or otherwise ejected from the gym.)

The
Six Basic Rules
of
Gym Etiquette

Rule One
DON'T BE A SLOB

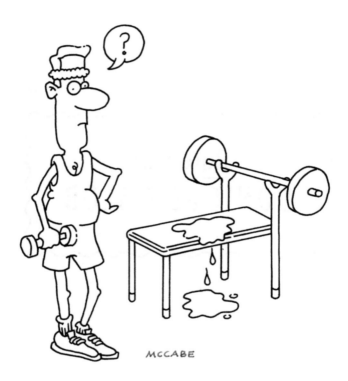

Wipe Up Sweat From the Equipment

Let's be clear about the topic of sweat at the gym. It's a good thing to sweat when you work out. Indeed, the whole point of working out is to work up a sweat. But, those who happen to sweat on the machines or the equipment need to wipe it up. It's the polite and sanitary thing to do.

People should always wipe the machines with a towel after they finish their workout. Just hope they don't leave their towels around afterward.

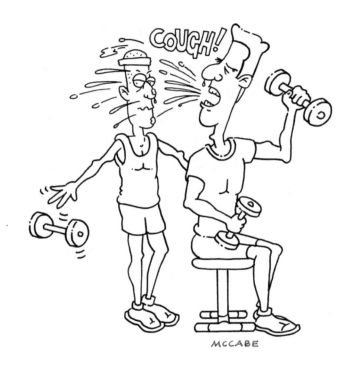

Cover Your Mouth
When You Cough or Sneeze

It goes without saying that no one should come to the gym (or any other public place where they will be in close proximity to others) if they are really sick or have a contagious condition. But, not everyone observes this rule, and even healthy people occasionally sneeze or cough—particularly during allergy season. So if and when people sneeze or cough at the gym, we hope they do the right thing and cover their mouths. If they forget, perhaps politely handing over some clean tissues will serve as an effective reminder.

Don't Leave Tissues Around

Gym-goers, like lots of people, seem to really love their tissues. But for goodness sake, people should not leave used tissues around the gym. There are few sights more disgusting than seeing a crumpled up tissue or napkin in the bottom of a gym machine cup-holder, particularly when you have already stuck your water bottle in there. It is equally gross to see tissues on the gym or locker room floor. People need to remember what their first grade teacher told them—used tissues belong in the wastepaper basket!

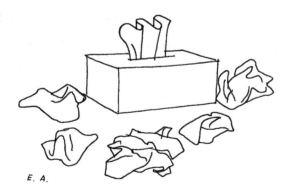

E. A.

Don't Leave Sweaty Towels Around

Nobody wants to touch a sweaty towel. Nor should anyone have to do so when they finally make it to the gym. So, don't leave used towels on the machines, the floor, the windowsill, the locker room bench, or any other place except the designated hamper or basket. Virtually every gym has a spot for depositing towels: all gym-goers need to do is to find it and use it.

This tip goes double for the egregious double towel violator I personally witnessed—the man who put one towel on the seat of an exercise bicycle and another

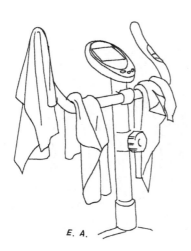 towel on its handles— and then proceeded to leave both of his sweaty towels on the bike after he was finished. Can you say double yuck?

E. A.

Don't Leave Water Bottles Around

When you are working out, there may be nothing more important than good hydration. Indeed, coaches strongly encourage athletes to drink lots of water when they exercise. With that in mind, almost everyone carries around a water bottle at the gym nowadays. But, not everyone seems to remember to put their empty water bottles in the proper receptacle. Be a decent gym-goer—don't force other people to deal with your water bottles; with any luck, you won't have to deal with theirs. Take your water bottles with you or toss them in the recycling bin.

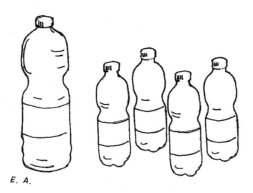

E. A.

Don't Leave Hair in the Sink or Shower

We don't like to see our own hair in the sink or the shower drain, so we certainly don't want to see someone else's hair there either. Yet, there's plenty of errant hair whirling around the gym, especially in the hairdryer area and on the shower floor. Everyone should take note of whether they left a clump of hair somewhere at the gym and do the polite thing: pick up the hair from wherever it fell and throw it out.

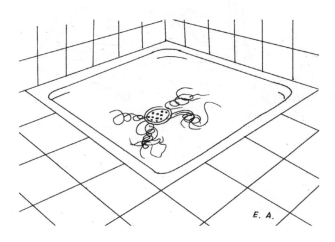

E. A.

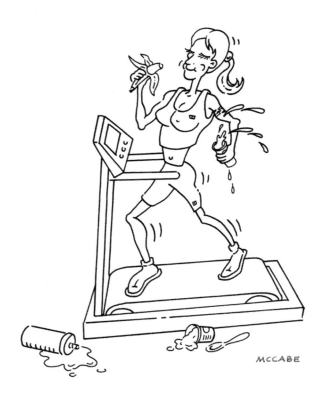

Don't Turn Workout Time Into Meal Time

Some gyms have a refreshment area. It's perfectly fine to eat there—in fact they probably want you to hang out, eat some fruit, chug some cold water, and do a wheat grass juice shot or two. But, some people don't seem to realize that eating in the rest of the gym is just plain inconsiderate and even a bit disgusting. No one wants to smell someone else's food, or see crumbs, yogurt splashes or wrappers on the machines or the windowsills.

Keep in mind that many gym-goers are dieting and therefore don't want to be exposed to bagels and breakfast sandwiches—we can't even believe people are eating them between sets. But, in any event, watching someone consume a meal on the gym floor just isn't appetizing. The gym floor should not be mistaken for a café, and no one should mistake workout time for meal time.

Don't Leave Reading Material Around

How many times have you gotten to a machine only to find a crumpled, sweaty magazine or newspaper draped over it? Maybe the folks who left these behind have someone to pick up after them at home, and there might even be people whose job it is to straighten up your gym, but it isn't possible for any gym to provide constant and instantaneous removal of people's detritus. Avid gym readers should remember to take their reading materials with them or to place them on the magazine rack for others to enjoy.

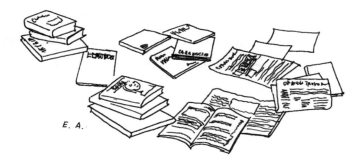

E. A.

Put Equipment Away After You Use It

This may be the most fundamental gym etiquette rule of all, and it's so simple yet is so often ignored. After people use weights or other gym equipment, they need to put the equipment back where it came from. All gyms have racks or hooks or other designated places to hold equipment. If people don't put the gym equipment back in the proper place, others will either trip on it and/or be unable to find it, which is both dangerous and frustrating.

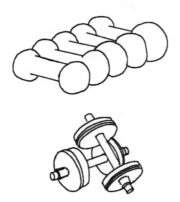

E. A.

Suggested responses to
A SLOB

Polite Response

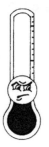

When You Are Mildly Annoyed

Excuse me. It's getting a little messy here. Would you mind being a little neater with your stuff? Many thanks.

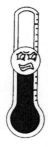

Slightly Rude Response

When You Are Very Irritated

*Dude, your stuff is in my way.
Could you please move it?*

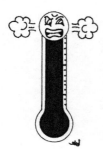

Very Rude Response

What You WISH You Could Say
When You Are Experiencing
Full-Scale Gym Rage

*Please, **please** get away from me,
you @#%&ing slob!*

Rule Two
DON'T BE A HOG

Don't Use an Adjacent Piece of Equipment As Your Personal Hanger

Sure, your mother always told you to hang up your things. What she might not have told you, however, is that the only proper place to hang up your coat (or other clothing) at the gym is on a coat rack or on the hook in your locker. At some gyms, it might also be okay to store your things neatly on an out-of-the-way windowsill, countertop, or shelf. But, one of the rudest things someone can do at any gym is to just

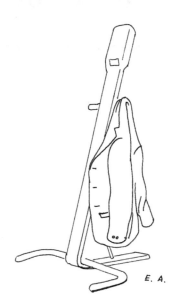

E. A.

throw their stuff onto an adjacent piece of equipment. Now the unsuspecting gym-goer who wants to use the machine that is covered with stuff is in the uncomfortable position of having to interrupt the offender's workout to ask them to move it. The alternative for such folks is to move it themselves: which never goes over very well. Polite gym-goers should avoid putting anyone else in that position, and keep their stuff out of the way.

If someone is planning to arrive and leave the gym in workout gear, it admittedly might be easier to forego the whole locker room thing. But if they do plan to bring their coat or workout bag with them to the gym floor, they need to make sure that there is an out-of-the-way place to neatly store the stuff.

Don't Hog a Popular Machine

It is a gym fact—some machines are more popular than others. Furthermore, during peak times, it can be difficult to get on even the not-so-popular machines. And even though many gyms post little signs asking patrons to observe a twenty minute limit if others are waiting, let's face it—everyone ignores those notices if they feel the need to go for more than twenty minutes. So, what is the solution? The only answer is for everyone to be reasonable. If someone is waiting for the machine, people should earnestly try to limit their time on that apparatus to 30 minutes or so.

If someone really wants to do a full hour of cardio, they should work out during off-peak times when the gym is relatively empty and/or pick a machine that has many duplicates. (They should keep in mind that, even if they feel like doing a full hour of cardio, many personal trainers would recommend they mix it up anyway.) The bottom line when it comes to using gym equipment is that everyone should do what they were taught to do in grade school: share and be fair.

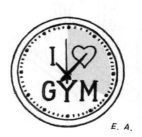

E. A.

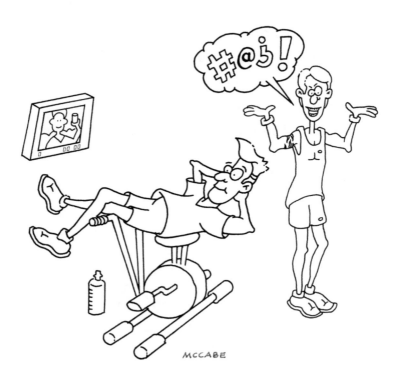

MCCABE

Don't Use a Piece of Equipment Just to Rest or Watch TV

It is difficult enough to wait politely for someone to get off a machine they are actually using for their workout. Now imagine how irritating it is to have to wait for someone to get off a machine they aren't actually using for their workout.

Maybe they're tired, and that exercise bicycle seat looked like a really comfy place to take a breather, but for the sake of everyone else at the gym, they should know that commandeering equipment as a place to relax is a big no-no. Gym equipment (including those all-inviting, cushioned stretching tables) should be reserved for workouts, not for rest stops, television breaks, or naps.

Don't Block the Mirrors

Gyms have mirrors for a reason. They enable gym-goers to check their exercise technique. Consequently, the gym is actually one of the few places where it is perfectly acceptable for people to stare at themselves in the mirror. All gym-goers should do their best to avoid walking or lingering in front of people who are working out in front of a mirror, especially in the middle of a set.

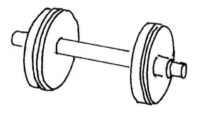

E. A.

Share the Bench in the Locker Room

There is a limited window of time, right after a gym-goer has returned to the locker room and is ready to get dressed (after a workout or post-workout shower), when they probably need the most space on the locker room bench. They need room to sit down so they can put shoes and socks on, and a place to put clothes and other belongings just for a short time while they get dressed. Somehow, that always seems to be exactly the same moment that someone else with a boatload of stuff and a locker right nearby wants to use the same bench.

To keep locker room frustration to a minimum, people need to avoid spreading their stuff out over the entire bench and should move some of it to make some space for their locker room neighbor. If this is done promptly, there will be no need for the new entrant to glare viciously, or even worse, to verbally berate the other person into moving his or her things. It actually helps when both people acknowledge the situation, try to accommodate each other's needs, and declare that there is no problem.

Don't Ask to "Just Work In" and Then Plan to Stay

There's nothing sneakier than a pretend-polite gym-goer. One of the most egregious examples of this is the "worker inner" who asks if he can "just work in" and allegedly use a given piece of gym equipment just between your sets. Inevitably, the worker inner not only works in but stays in for the entire workout. It's pretty annoying.

If the gym is super-crowded and someone absolutely feels the need to "work in" to your workout, then that person should do it quickly, vacate the machine, and make sure they aren't holding up your workout.

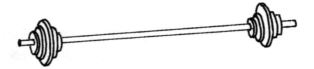

E. A.

Choose One TV to Watch While You Are Working Out

Many modern gyms have multiple television screens in front of the cardio machines and a sound system that allows exercisers to plug headphones in to hear the broadcast. Even when employing the most sophisticated sound equipment, it is a scientific fact that it is only possible to tune into one station at a time. However, in every gym with TVs, there will always be a handful of greedy gym-goers who insist on monopolizing multiple TV screens at once.

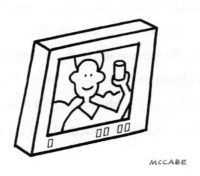

MCCABE

There are, in fact, two types of TV-watching gym-goers. A TV-watcher is either a channel-setter or a passive watcher. A channel-setter feels the need to make sure the channel of his or her choice is displayed on the television that is most directly in front of the machine that he or she plans to use. Etiquette suggests that the channel-setter wave to others within view of that particular television to confirm that it is OK with them to change the channel. This is a nice practice, but it can be annoying at the same time. The passive-watcher rarely says no anyway, and when his or her workout is interrupted by a channel-setter's frantic waving, it frequently scares the daylights out of that person because he or she is actually listening to music through headphones and staring into space, only occasionally checking out the television screens. (As an aside, I have often marveled at those who forego music to work out to channels like CNBC: indeed, I have no idea how the CNBC-types achieve workout flow while viewing dull, and often depressing, facts about the economy.)

Channel-setters should limit their waving appropriately and simply point up to the TV they wish to program. There is no need to get each and every individual's full attention, particularly if someone is not looking at the screen anyway. If it is that difficult to get someone to focus on that screen, chances are they do not care if it is changed.

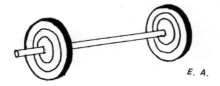

E. A.

Don't Expect Others to Spot You All Day

People shouldn't ask someone to spot them and expect that person to stay with them for the duration of their workout. It is one thing to ask for occasional help, and another thing to request an assistant for the whole workout. Remember, other people are at the gym to exercise too, and not just there as volunteer personal trainers. It is okay for someone to ask for help if he or she needs it, but it certainly isn't right to take advantage of people who are just being nice by taking up all their workout time.

Don't Mark Your Territory to Save Equipment and Then Leave the Room

Someone sees an open machine. He knows he wants to use it. But, polite gym-goers know that you either use or lose it. Under no circumstance should gym-goers leave their sneakers, newspaper, locker key, water bottle, towel, underwear or anything else on a select machine, then leave the room to do their business, and expect that machine to sit idle. Animals mark their territory: people at the gym shouldn't. They should remember those embarrassing grade school moments when they tried to sit down and another kid said that "seat was saved" (even though there wasn't another kid in sight). Gym-goers who engage in obvious machine-marking behavior are likely offending everyone around them and should demonstrate maturity by refraining from taking measures to "save" machines.

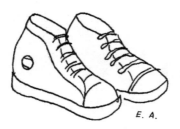

E. A.

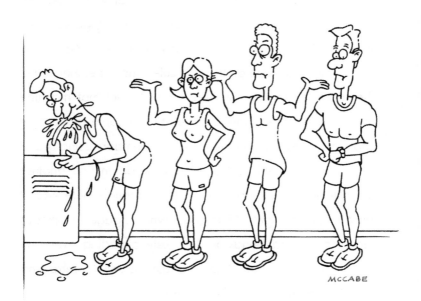

Don't Hog the Water Fountain

Despite the popularity of bottled water, most gyms still have water fountains. Gym-goers who use the water from the fountain to fill up their super-sized water bottle should step aside if there are others behind who just want a quick sip. And it should go without saying that no one should have to see someone put their saliva or gum into the water fountain. It's a public fountain; not a private watering hole!

Don't Linger on a Machine When You Are Finished

Let's assume you have waited patiently for a particular piece of equipment. You haven't bugged the person in any way, haven't asked them when they will be done, but instead just have quietly stayed nearby and otherwise occupied yourself. The person finally finishes, and you are relieved, psyched up, and ready to go. Then, what could possibly be more annoying than to have that person take forever to get off the machine? It's nothing less than remarkable when people do this. Instead of quickly wiping their sweat off the machine, removing their articles, and moving off the equipment, they stand there for what seems like an inordinate amount of time, stretching, recovering, chatting, drinking and doing whatever else they feel like at a glacial pace. Their selfish attitude is transparent: What do they care? They are finished with their workout.

Nobody should engage in selfish behavior like this at the gym. When a gym-goer finishes with any piece of equipment, whether it is a cardio machine or a workout bench, they need to clear their stuff up and go rather than just lingering there.

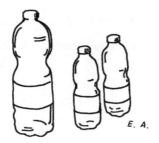

E. A.

Suggested responses to
A HOG

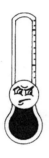

Polite Response

When You Are Mildly Annoyed

Pardon me, but especially since we are in close quarters here, would you mind sharing your workout space? Much appreciated.

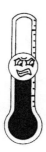

Slightly Rude Response

When You Are Very Irritated

Dude, you can't keep that equipment all to yourself. The rest of us need a turn.

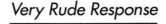

Very Rude Response

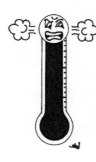

What You WISH You Could Say When You Are Experiencing Full-Scale Gym Rage

This isn't your personal gym, you @#%&ing hog! You need to share that equipment with the rest of us.

Rule Three

DON'T BE A
SPACE INVADER

Respect Other People's Workout Space

As part of driver's ed classes in high school, they showed us films to promote safe driving. We were told to keep a "space cushion" around our vehicle whenever possible: I can clearly remember one of the films depicting a cartoon of a car on a highway with these massive horizontal and vertical arrows coming out of it to form a big space cushion around the entire vehicle. Since my high school days, much has been published about the importance of respecting the "personal space" of others. (That, by the way, is precisely what they now tell preschoolers to do when they simply can't seem to stop hugging, poking, and otherwise touching their friends while waiting in line.)

Everyone who works out in a public gym should think of themselves like a vehicle surrounded by a big space cushion and stay as far away as possible from others' personal space. That means, for example, keeping arms and legs and other body parts within the confines of the particular piece of cardio equipment being used. While this might seem like an obvious way to

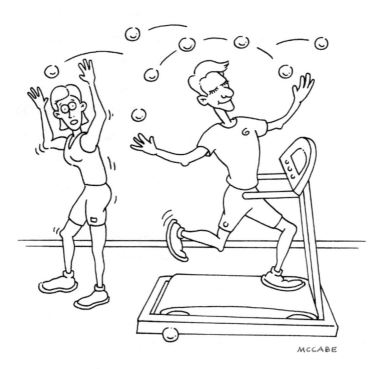

MCCABE

behave at the gym, let me assure you that it isn't obvious to all gym-goers. Indeed, I have personally witnessed a "conductor" who, while on the stairmill, moves her arms wildly around so that they extend far into the airspace of the adjacent machine. I have also observed a "Rockette®" who kicks her legs widely and wildly from side to side while on the Stairmaster®. Similarly, I have even marveled at the sight of a juggler, who rapidly juggles three balls while he runs on the treadmill. Despite this being a truly impressive, even circus-like feat, you might imagine how annoying his workout routine was to neighboring treadmillers, who clearly couldn't stand his arms and juggling balls in their faces, and feared being pelted by one of the hard rubber balls.

No Loud Conversations With Trainers or Other People Working Out

Not only do fellow gym-goers have zero desire to hear other people's phone conversations, the truth is that most of the time, they don't want to be privy to any conversations at the gym, including other people's conversations with their trainers.

Not to sound like an elementary school teacher, but while inside the gym, people need to remember to use their "indoor voice" so they don't annoy or interrupt fellow gym-goers with their loud or raucous conversations. People need to keep in mind at all times that it's a gym, not an outdoor playground—and certainly not a bar where it is appropriate for anyone to be calling out orders and getting the attention of everyone in the room.

No Dropping
or Throwing Weights

When dropped or tossed onto the ground, weights make a thunderous noise. The noise and vibrations from a dropped weight can be distracting and even scary to others. There is no need to make a ruckus at the gym. People should be in good enough shape and courteous enough to others at the gym to simply place the weight down.

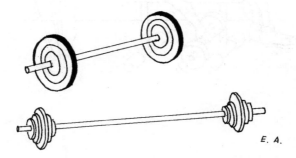

E. A.

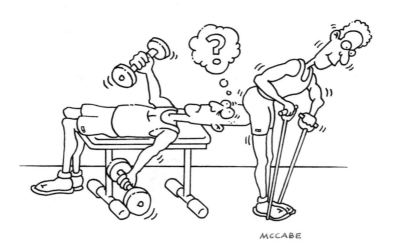

Mind the Body Odor

We have already established that no one wants to see, hear, or feel someone else in their workout space at the gym. Then it shouldn't surprise you that they don't want to smell someone else either—ever! That includes being subjected to someone else's heavy cologne or perfume. People simply need to keep all of their smells to themselves! Everyone should wear appropriate and clean clothing, use deodorant, and not wait too long to shower; in short, they need to do what is necessary to avoid smelling bad at the gym. And just to be on the safe side, everybody should be reminded to keep a space cushion around themselves at all times.

No Excessive Grunting or Exhaling

Some people are just noisier than others. That is true whether we are referring to people talking, eating, having sex, or working out (and not necessarily in that order). But, for the sake of all gym-goers, everyone needs to monitor the sounds that are coming out of their bodies when they are working out. They just shouldn't allow themselves to grunt, exhale, scream or otherwise make noises to the point of being disgusting or disruptive to others. We would appreciate it if everyone would just keep all aspects of their workout to themselves—including their personal soundtrack.

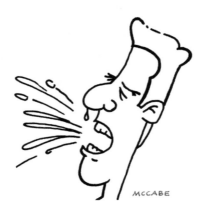

MCCABE

Don't Use, Move, or Take Anyone Else's Stuff

The most egregious gym behavior of all, of course, is stealing from others. And yet, people seem to get their belongings stolen all the time at gyms. I would like to think people are just tired and not paying attention when they pick up someone else's similar-looking iPod® or jacket. Whether this behavior is intentional or unintentional, however, it must be eliminated.

Similarly, unless it really and truly cannot be avoided, people shouldn't even move anyone else's stuff. It is not their place to tidy up the gym. Gym-goers expect to find their half-filled water bottles where they left them. Moreover, unless they have rudely abandoned a particular item, they don't want anyone to touch or use their belongings. People should refrain from moving or using their fellow gym-goers' stuff.

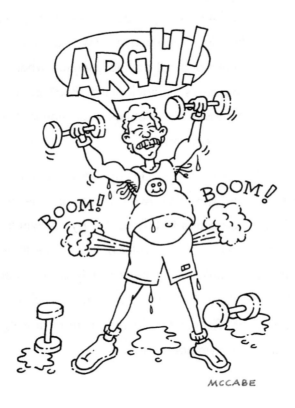

Watch the Gas

I am sure there is a medical reason for this, but at the risk of being crass, it is a fact that when you move around, you are somehow more inclined to pass gas. And of course, the whole goal of working out is to move your body around. So let me be so brave as to just come out and say what many others have observed throughout the years: while they are exercising, people frequently feel the need to pass gas. The polite thing, my friends, is not to keep working out, let one rip, and pretend it was someone else who did it. This principle applies equally in the sauna (or another enclosed space), if you are lucky enough to have one in your gym. People need to take serious steps to prevent their gas from seeping into another's personal space. If they feel the need, they should walk away, find a bathroom or a hall somewhere and spare their fellow gym-goers the annoyance and disgust. Well, somebody had to say it!

Suggested responses to
A SPACE-INVADER

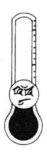

Polite Response

When You Are Mildly Annoyed

I'm feeling a little crowded.
Could you please give me
a little more space here? Thanks.

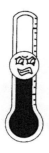

Slightly Rude Response

When You Are Very Irritated

Dude, you are in my face. Could you move out of my workout space?

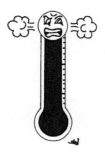

Very Rude Response

What You WISH You Could Say When You Are Experiencing Full-Scale Gym Rage

Get the @#%& away from me, you space invader!

Rule Four
DON'T BE A
SUPER-TALKER

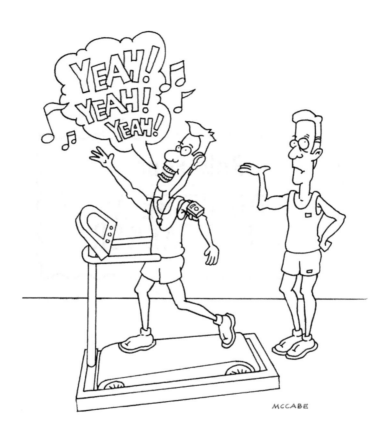

Don't Sing Out Loud

It has been said that people who listen to music while working out are more likely to exercise regularly than those who don't. Music definitely can make a workout more quick-moving, energetic and enjoyable. But, sometimes, people who listen to music while they work out get so into their music, they simply forget where they are and actually start singing out loud. For the most part, they don't even realize they are doing it. But, other people at the gym (particularly those who aren't listening to music at that moment) are acutely aware of the noise and painfully aware of the fact that these casual gym singers are no Lady Gaga. Furthermore, even if someone is using an iPod®, the music shouldn't be blasting so loudly through headphones that others can hear it. The key for these people is to remember that, when they are in the gym, they are in a public place. Gym-goers should always keep their music and their singing to themselves.

Don't Tell Anyone Else How to Work Out

Unless someone is actually employed by the gym as a trainer or has been specifically solicited for their advice on the subject, people should never try to tell anyone else at the gym how to work out. It is not their place to do so. In fact, no matter how good the intentions are, it is just not cool to scrutinize or comment on another person's technique.

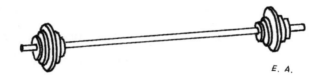

E. A.

In General, Don't Be a Chatterbox at the Gym

Some people may be bored or lonely, with plenty of time on their hands, but they shouldn't assume others are in the same boat. Many of us really struggle to find the time to work out, and when we do get to the gym, we have no time to waste. Some folks need to work out efficiently or they simply will not have the time to complete their session. Before anyone strikes up a lengthy conversation with any fellow gym-goers, they should keep in mind that some people might be on a tight timetable. This doesn't mean people shouldn't be cordial to everyone at the gym, but gym-goers should try and discern whether the person they're chatting with seems eager to continue the conversation.

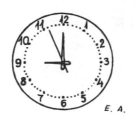

E. A.

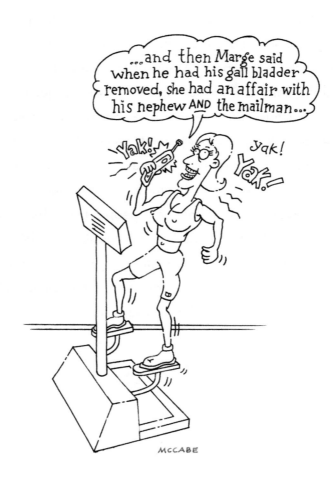

Don't Talk on Your Cell Phone

The gym floor is a noisy place, so if you were going to be so impolite as to talk on the phone at the gym, it follows that you would need to talk very loudly for the person on the other end to hear you clearly. But, luckily the workout area of the gym is not the place for phone conversations. Indeed, most gyms acknowledge this with written signs that implore gym-goers to either refrain from any cell phone conversations (the cell phone-with-the-red-line-through-it depiction also gets the point across) or to keep them extremely limited.

Unless there is truly an emergency in their life underway (and then, I'm not exactly sure why they would be at the gym working out anyway), people should not even tempt themselves by bringing their cell phones onto the gym floor. The fact is that no one at the gym wants to hear telephone conversations. If there is a need to be in communication with the outside world during a workout (and those of us who work and/or have children frequently do), sending an email or a text message is a far less obtrusive way to go.

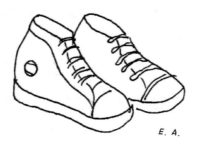

E. A.

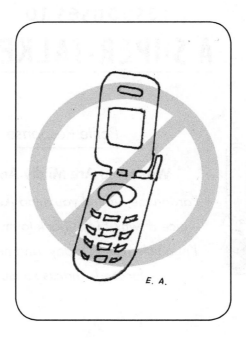

E. A.

Suggested responses to
A SUPER-TALKER

Polite Response

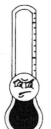

When You Are Mildly Annoyed

Pardon me, would you mind [keeping your voice down/if I get back to my workout]? I'm a little rushed today, and need to keep focused. Thanks so much.

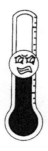

Slightly Rude Response

When You Are Very Irritated

Man, do you ever stop talking?
Don't be such a chatterbox.

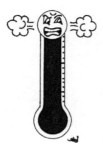

Very Rude Response

What You WISH You Could Say
When You Are Experiencing
Full-Scale Gym Rage

Shut the @#%& up,
you annoying super-talker!"

Rule Five
DON'T BE A GROUCH

Be Polite

Everyone needs to remain polite to fellow gym-goers—even if they are doing something that is very annoying. Thus, even if someone is really disappointed not to have access to a particular machine because another person is on it, they need to stay calm. Similarly, even if someone witnesses people leaving their personal items and trash around the gym, they have to keep their cool. Reacting rudely will just make the situation worse. Furthermore, even if someone hogs an entire bench in the locker room, everyone will have a much better day if all involved keep their cool.

The gym isn't a place to forget your manners: indeed, it is one of the most important places in which to display good manners. Just because people are rushing to or around the gym doesn't mean they can cut people off, slam doors, or forget to say "please" and "thank you." Spread good karma at the gym with good manners at all times.

Finally, everyone knows that is impolite to stare at others. That goes doubly at the gym. Staring is just plain rude, and it makes other people feel uncomfortable. People should focus on themselves and on having the best workout possible. It certainly doesn't help your workout to stare at or compete with others at your gym.

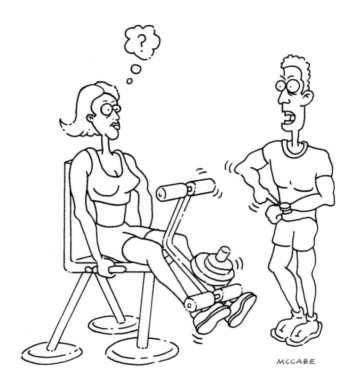

Don't Interrupt

Some people bark at others in the guise of asking them how long they "have left" on a particular machine. Yes, there are folks who can't help being grumpy about this issue. We get it: they want that person to get off right now, but asking another gym-goer how much time they have left and then reacting disapprovingly does nothing but spread "gymisery." Barring an emergency, no one should be interrupting anyone who is in the middle of exercising. It's rude, crotchety, and totally kills the flow. Everyone should avoid this type of "exercisus interruptus" and learn to leave fellow gym-goers in peace!

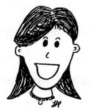
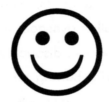
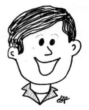

Be Pleasant

In an ideal world, each gym-goer would be surrounded by a river of positive energy and have the ability to focus singularly on his or her workout. Unfortunately, it is not an ideal world for gym-goers (maybe this book will change that?). Indeed, there are plenty of miserable people marching around the gym who occasionally suck the life-force right out of other gym-goers.

Even when they are in a rush, people need to be pleasant and cordial to others at the gym—no matter what. The gym is a shared and special place that people visit to look and feel better; gym-goers need to respect its sanctity by doing their best to preserve and promote positive energy at the gym.

Suggested responses to

A GROUCH

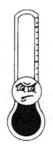

Polite Response

When You Are Mildly Annoyed

I understand you would like to [use this piece of equipment/get to your workout], but please, let's do what we can to keep things as pleasant as possible here.

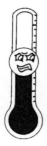

Slightly Rude Response

When You Are Very Irritated

Don't be such a bummer.
We're all just trying to get
our workouts in.

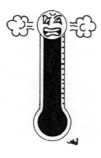

Very Rude Response

What You WISH You Could Say
When You Are Experiencing
Full-Scale Gym Rage

@#%& you, you miserable grouch!

Rule Six

DON'T BE AN EXHIBITIONIST

Wear Appropriate Workout Clothing

I have yet to work out at gym that enforces a strict dress code. But, I don't think that's a crazy idea. How many times have you seen more than you ever wanted to see of a fellow gym-goer because he or she was wearing a workout outfit that was just plain too small or cut way too low?

There you are trying hard to focus on your workout—and trying not to think mean thoughts. But, you can't help asking yourself why that incredibly hairy man working out in front of you insists on wearing tight, tiny shorts with slits up the sides and a matching sleeveless tank top. And you can't help but ponder how the woman with the protruding stomach has the nerve to wear a halter top you wouldn't be caught dead in. Finally, despite your best efforts to ignore others, you ask yourself why yet another woman at your gym felt the need to wear a thong under her gym pants when she was planning to do lunges across the length of the gym floor.

Dressing properly for the gym shouldn't be difficult. A short sleeve shirt that's not too tight and a decent pair of gym shorts or pants that covers the bellybutton (and otherwise provides ample coverage), coupled with proper footwear, will do the trick every time.

And the Pilates folks (who aren't allowed to wear footwear on the Pilates machines themselves) should remember to wear shoes when walking to and from their Pilates workout. Walking around any part of the gym in bare feet is off-limits, no matter what type of exercise we are discussing.

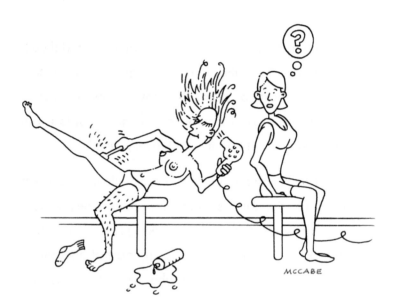

Don't Unnecessarily Parade Around the Locker Room Naked

Some people might be comfortable prancing around the locker room completely naked for an extended period of time while they blow dry and style their hair, check the messages on their Blackberry®, and apply body lotion—but not everyone is that evolved. Of course the locker room is a fully acceptable place in which to change clothes, but people need to respect others and not make them unduly uncomfortable with their rampant nakedness.

The fact is that, barring the occasional pervert, nobody at the gym wants to look at someone else naked. It doesn't matter whether they are in good shape or in bad shape. If they are in really good shape, other people don't want to see them naked because it will just make them feel bad. And, if they are out-of-shape, people really don't want to see them naked, especially in the harsh light of the locker room. When it comes to showering, changing and doing their business in the locker room, people should be quick and discreet. Also, it goes without saying that no one should ever sit down naked on a locker room bench without at least putting a towel down first!

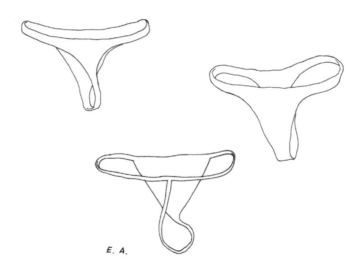

E. A.

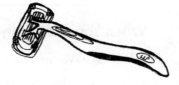

Suggested
responses to
AN EXHIBITIONIST

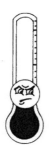

Polite Response

When You Are Mildly Annoyed

Pardon me. Would you mind covering up a bit? It makes the rest of us a little uncomfortable. We really appreciate it.

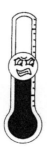

Slightly Rude Response

When You Are Very Irritated

*Dude, what's with the
excessive nakedness?
Cover it up like the rest of us.*

Very Rude Response

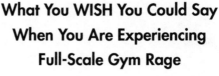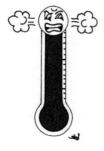

What You WISH You Could Say
When You Are Experiencing
Full-Scale Gym Rage

*None of us want to see that much
of your naked, exhibitionist self.
Give us a @#%&ing break and
wrap a towel around yourself!*

Finally

HEAD TO THE SHOWERS

Conquering Your Gym Rage:

Unfortunately, even with some subtle (and not-so-subtle) hints, some of your fellow gym-goers may not get the message. What's a workout-lover to do? Here are six non-confrontational ways to turn down your gym rage, lower your blood pressure, and keep other's bad behavior from turning a healthy activity into a toxic one:

- Take a deep breath and then crank up the volume on your iPod®.

- Move to another piece of equipment or part of the gym.

- Take a break and head for the juice bar.

- Go make a massage appointment.

- Head to the showers.

- Start planning your home gym.